A SURVIVAL GUIDE: THE FIRST <u>30</u> DAYS OF PARALYSIS

By Matt Gustafson

© Copyright 2020 - Move Forward 365

Dedication

I'd like to dedicate this book to...

My mom and dad

Acknowledgments

I'd like to thank...

Debora Pinheiro Gustafson

Scott Gustafson

Marc and Jane Gustafson

Jereme Gilbert

Cameron Gross

Robbie Parks

Brian Muscarella

Taylor Wingate

Table of Contents

Chapter 1

Introduction

The purpose of this book is to provide easy access to information in a positive, motivational manner when facing the first 30 days of paralysis. This book focuses on helping the person and family that has been affected by paralysis. This book was not written to be directed towards people who are paralyzed with a specific spinal cord injury (SCI) or use a particular type of wheelchair. This book sometimes uses examples based on the author's own experiences and personal specific paralysis. The author is not a paid sponsor nor endorser of products; they are being shown as examples and further reference materials only. This book will cover the following topics: Introduction, Before Leaving Rehabilitation, Adaptability and Mobility Equipment, Living Space Adaptability and Mobility, Medical supplies and Catheters, Health and Nutrition, Bowel Management, Healthy Body Weight, Vitamins and Supplements, Pressure Ulcers – Signs of, Preventing and Healing, Infection and Complications, Mental Health – Coping and Adjustment, Don't Panic! You WILL fall! (How to recover from a fall), Exercise and Preventing Injury, Playing Adaptive Sports, Social Meetings and Relationships, Choosing and Starting A New Career, Traveling, Clinical Research (stem cells), New Technology, and

Exoskeleton Suits, and much more helpful information and links located in the appendix.

Before leaving rehabilitation

This section covers some of the crucial questions that one should be asking oneself, the information that one needs to know, and research before leaving one's rehabilitation center. Some examples of questions are below. I hope these questions give you an idea as to what one will need to be thinking about and planning for before leaving the rehabilitation center. Not all items below will be suited to one's specific needs but will cover the majority of them. Take a look at the questions below, answer them, and then add additional items that one might need explaining.

- What kind of adaptability and mobility equipment will need to order before leaving rehab?
- Does the rehabilitation center have a fulltime person that can help patients with obtaining adaptability and mobility equipment?
- Where to find help with adaptability and mobility equipment if the rehabilitation center doesn't have a liaison that does for its patients?
- What are the names of the local adaptability and mobility equipment suppliers?

- Will the doorways in my residence need to be modified for accessibility?
- Will a wheelchair ramp be needed for accessibility?
- Will handrails need to be installed in the bathroom and shower area?
- Will a shower head extension hose be needed for the shower?
- Will the bed frame height or bed's mattress need to be changed in the bedroom?
- Will a shower chair be needed for the shower or tub?
- Will a toilet chair be needed?
- Is the bathroom accessible by wheelchair?
- Will a family member or a home nurse be needed to help me daily with medical needs, cooking, and cleaning?
- Will things throughout the home need to be lowered for easy reaching?
- Who will be ordering my monthly medical supplies?
- What will be the mode of transportation to and from additional rehab and doctor's appointments?
- Is the current vehicle accessible by a wheelchair?
- Will one be able to drive a vehicle?

After one has read through all the above questions, I can imagine that there are more questions that one might have that need to be answered and researched. I would start by making a list of all the problems that one might think will need answers for, then talk to other patients, one's rehabilitation specialist, doctor, and nurse, then search the internet for additional possible answers. It would be best to have all one's questions answered before leaving the rehabilitation center. Getting answers to these questions will alleviate all the unnecessary headaches in the future.

Chapter 2

Adaptability and Mobility Equipment

When starting to think, research about the specific equipment that one will need for one's specific adaptability and mobility needs, it is best to think about the larger pieces of equipment that one will need first. What type of wheelchair will one be needing a manual or specialty motorized wheelchair? Will one want a folding or rigid frame manual wheelchair? Will the wheelchair to have tilting or standing or both capabilities? What will be the best wheelchair cushion for you? What type of shower chair will one be needing? What kinds of grab bars will one need to be installed, and in what locations? Will the grab bars need to be installed by a professional? Will one need a body lift for the home? Will one need a specialty mattress?

To determine what type of wheelchair, wheelchair cushion, and other adaptability and mobility items will one need, I would recommend talking to one's rehabilitation therapist, nurse, or center coordinator to find out if they have a seating clinic at the rehabilitation center. This seating clinic room should have many different types of wheelchairs, cushions that one can try out before making the final decision. If the rehabilitation center does not have a seating clinic or a primary contact person to answer one's seating questions, one can try to contact a support group or local wheelchair supply company. They would be able to help figure out all the necessary adaptability and mobility equipment that one will need in the home.

It is best to start researching this as soon as possible due to the amount of time it takes to get this equipment ordered and delivered. The one thing that I learned was to talk first with one's therapist there at the facility to see if they are aware of any well-known adaptability and mobility equipment companies in one's area. One could then can use the internet to do more research on these companies. One can also reach out to other patients there at the rehabilitation center to ask them if they know of any local adaptability and mobility equipment suppliers. When shopping for adaptability and mobility equipment for oneself, it is best to locate multiple suppliers. This way, one will be able to not only compare what equipment is available through each supplier, but the costs of the equipment, shipping cost, and the amount of time it will take to have the equipment delivered to the residence. Before making the equipment purchase or purchases, another significant consideration to take into account is if the supplier to purchase the equipment from would also be the one who would be making future repairs to the equipment when needed. If the supplier is not the company that would be making repairs to the equipment in the future, this might mean that one would be without equipment for a while. A situation that one would not want to find oneself.

Here is an example, I once had an axle pin on my manual wheelchair break late one Friday evening after returning home from having dinner with my family. The axle pin broke due to three years of normal wear, tear and use. So, I immediately got on the internet and started searching for wheelchair part suppliers that had next day air or two-day shipping. I was only able to locate one supplier that had two-day shipping available and could tell me if they had the part in inventory. Until the replacement axle pin arrived, I had to move around the house very cautiously so that the wheel wouldn't fall off my chair with me in it. Rule of thumb, when one has a manual wheelchair axle break due to normal wear, it is best to go ahead and replace both axle pins at the same time and keep one of the old axle pins as a backup for emergency use only.

The final consideration for choosing an adaptability and mobility equipment supplier to purchase from is whether they accept one's health insurance as payment, have a payment plan, or only accept credit cards or cash for payment.

Here is a recap of the questions that one might need to find answers for when purchasing the adaptive and mobility equipment for one's daily living:

- Who to contact that can help obtain the necessary adaptability and mobility equipment?
- What are the names of local medical supply companies from whom to purchase necessary adaptability and mobility equipment?
- What form of payment or health insurance will these adaptability and mobility equipment supply companies accept?
- What will be the delivery options and time frame of the delivery required for the adaptability and mobility equipment?
- Will, the company that is selling the adaptability and mobility equipment be making any future repair to equipment if needed?
- Does this company have professional installers to install grab bars?

Living Space Adaptability and Mobility

When it comes to accessibility and mobility in the home, the height of furniture, and the amount of floor space is vital. You will probably need to have many things adjusted in height, moved around in the home for one to be able to maneuver around in a wheelchair daily. The bathroom and kitchen are rooms that will need the most focus. Let's start with the bathroom since this room will probably need more adjustments than any other place in the house. Is the bathroom accessible by wheelchair? Is the floor space of the bathroom large enough for one to move around in the wheelchair? Is there enough space to make safe transfers to and from the wheelchair to the toilet and the shower chair? If the bathroom is not large enough for mobility and transferring, one might have to seek professional help to make some adaptability adjustments to this room. Below is an image of a fully accessible bathroom with a roll-in shower with a grab bar and a toilet with grab bars on both sides. There are some accessible bathroom diagrams and other examples of grab bars and shower chairs located in the appendix. One can also consult the ADA (Americans with Disabilities Act) website, ADA.gov for suitable floor space, vanity height, grab grip measurements, and more detailed bathroom layouts.

If the bathroom is large enough to move safely around, let's now start thinking about reachability. Reachability is the actual height or distance that someone is physically able to reach something without using a grabber tool. Are all the things in the bathroom physically reachable?

Will the shower head need to be lowered, or can a shower head extension hose be used? Who will be installing the shower head extension? Will a suction cup shower caddy for shampoo, soap and other shower necessities be needed? Will a non-slip shower mat for the shower or tub be required? Will a shower chair or stool be required?

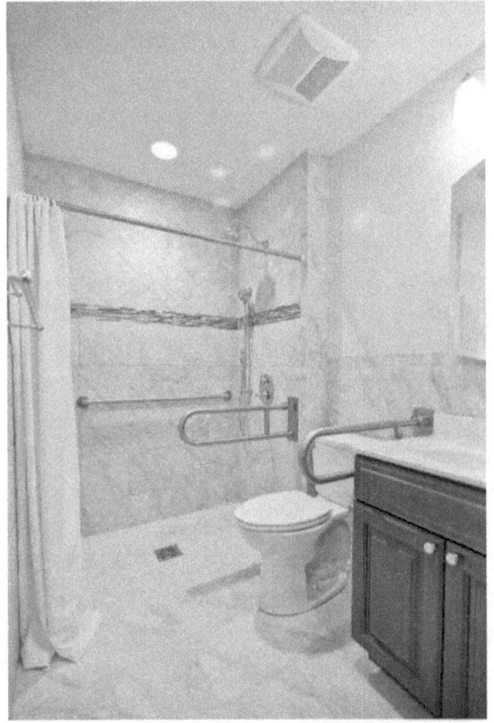

Now that we have covered the bathroom let's talk about the kitchen. In the kitchen, are food items low enough for one's physical reach? Are the power outlets reachable? Can the appliances be easily plugged into the outlets? Is the microwave easy to access? Is the refrigerator easy to open, reach an item, and then close again? Are the sink, stovetop, and oven easy, safe to use? The sink, stovetop, oven are all things that can be costly to upgrade to be more accessible. One will most likely need to seek professional help to get these items modified to be able to use. The sink's lower cabinet can be cut and modified to bring the sink closer. The stovetop and oven might have to be replaced altogether for a unit that is a more accessible design model. Consider the overall cost of these modifications.

Now let's focus on the bedroom and the other rooms of the house that might need some necessary modifications. Is the height of the bed low enough to be able to make a safe transfer? Will the bed frame need to be modified? Are there other pieces of furniture that will need to be changed? Is there enough floor space to be able to maneuver safely around in the home in a wheelchair? For example, before I left my rehabilitation center, I had my brother measure all the heights of all the furniture that I would be possibly transferring to like the living room couch or any chair and the bed in my bedroom. This way, I would know in advance what furniture I would need to be modified so that I could make an excellent transfer to them. I ended up having to lower my bed frame by three inches, the living room couch and chair would not need to be changed, but I would have to move them around to make more floor space and the room more maneuverable.

Chapter 3

Medical Supplies and Catheters

Before leaving the rehabilitation center, you need to know the answers to the following questions about one's medical supplies. Where will one be getting all the required monthly medical supplies? How will they be delivered to the residence? How many shipping days will the order take to arrive? How will the medical supplies be billed? When I was at my rehabilitation center, a nurse made sure that I knew how to use a catheter, and that was it. There was no one at my rehabilitation center to come to talk to me about the local medical supply companies that would be available to help me with my necessary monthly medical supply needs.

I asked my rehabilitation doctor about all the things that I would need to use daily from the type of catheter, gloves, surgical gel, iodine pads, briefs, underpads for my bed, and suppositories. Since I knew that I would be on disability for a while, I decided to research the difference in using my health insurance to pay for my medical supplies versus paying for them with my credit card. I was able to locate a medical supply company that would not only ship the medical supplies directly to my residence, allow me to charge supplies to a credit card, but also had free shipping. I also ordered some of my medical supplies through Amazon.com, but this was not always the cheapest source. The option of my ordering my medical supplies turned out to be a much less expensive option than having the medical supply company bill my health insurance. Until I can get back to working full-time at a company with excellent health insurance, this is my cheapest option when purchasing the necessary medical supplies that I will need each month. Now, I know that each person will not have this option of using a credit card in paying for their medical supplies, so this is very important to research all of one's available options. If one can prevent it, you don't want to have to limit oneself to just one medical supply company because they are the only one that will accept one's health insurance or that they are the only one that will take credit cards. It is best to have more than one medical supply company that one can reach out to for one's supplies. And the reason for this is because medical supply companies are not always the manufacturers; they are just a supplier. So, they might run out of the catheters or briefs or any other medical supplies that one will need to order when you need them. Therefore, it is best to have a primary medical supplier, a backup medical supplier that you can order from when in a bind. For example, I once lost track of the number of medical supplies that I had at home, needed to order some catheters very quickly. Unfortunately, the medical supply company that I would typically order from was out of the catheters that I needed, and they couldn't get them to my house in the amount of time that I needed them.

Here is a recap of the questions that you need to find answers for when purchasing one's daily medical supplies:

- What are the required monthly medical supplies?
- What medical supply company will be supplying the monthly medical supplies?
- Are these medical supply companies local or located in another state?
- What forms of payment or health insurance will this company accept?
- What will be the delivery options and time frame of the delivery of the monthly medical supplies?

Catheters are a necessity for daily living with paralysis, so let's start by talking about them.

IMPORTANT: Don't leave the hospital or rehabilitation center without a prescription from one's doctor for catheters!!!

I made this mistake, had to stress about how I would be able to purchase catheters without a prescription. In my state, North Carolina, one cannot buy catheters without a prescription. I disagree with this law since a catheter is not a medicine, but a daily necessity to live as a paralyzed person, but it's the law in my state.

There are many different types of catheters, the types of catheter tips, the coating that they can come with, and the way they can come packaged. I will be covering some of the differences in the catheter supplies that I have purchased. Then we will move on to the different types of briefs and other pieces of equipment that I have bought or used from my own experience. The first thing I am going to cover is what's called intermittent catheters. The definition of an intermittent catheter (IC) is the insertion and removal of a catheter several times daily to empty the bladder. The purpose of catheterization is to drain the bladder that is not correctly unloading due to paralysis or a surgical procedure. Intermittent catheters are catheters that I use daily every three to four hours to empty my bladder manually. Intermittent catheters come in many different materials, kit configurations, tip types, coatings, lengths, and diameters.

Intermittent catheters produced from the following materials: PVC, Silicone, and red rubber latex. PVC catheters are stiff and not very flexible, silicone catheters have medium flexibility, and the red rubber latex catheters are the most flexible and softest of them all. Latex catheters may not be an option for some.

The catheterization kits available for daily usage or usage when traveling is called a closed system intermittent catheter or no-touch catheters. They consist of a catheter that comes attached to a reservoir urine collection bag where the catheter is pre-lubricated. The catheter is sealed inside the urine collection bag until one inserts it into the urethra. These enclosed systems or no-touch catheter kits are suitable for traveling, ease of catheterization when not in a calm environment, and they also keep the chances of a urinary tract infection to a minimal. The only downside to these enclosed or no-touch kits is that they are very costly for daily usage over buying the individual supplies separately in bulk. Obtaining the medical supplies in bulk for home usage or travel, one can save lots of money but also means that when you pack for travel, one will have to prepare more in this area. When I travel and use bulk medical supplies, I package my catheter kits in zip lock bags for each use. I plan out my trip based on the number of days of my trip times the number of catheterizations that I will need to complete. I can then make up the number of kits that I will need plus a few extras for backup. By making up my kits for travel or daily usage when not at home, I can save lots of medical expenses over time. So, if you have time or don't mind making up one's catheter kits, this is the way to go. But, if you don't have time to make one's catheterization kits, want to save time, research the best catheterization kit for oneself, and their costs before making the purchase.

Now let's talk about the types of tips that are available for intermittent catheters. There are straight, Coude (pronounced as kuday), olive, introducer, round, open, cone, and whistle tip catheters. The straight tip catheter is the most commonly used, are mostly disposable, and can come pre-lubricated to ease the process of catheterization. One can get straight tip catheters just by themselves pre-lubricated or in a closed system intermittent, also called no-touch catheter bag kits.

The Coude tip catheter is a catheter that has a bent elbow (30 degrees) like tip shape. If a person has blockage because of the prostate or the urethra contracts and becomes blocked, the Coude catheter can easily bypass this blockage. In contrast, the straight catheter just might not work as with the straight catheter, one can also get the Coude catheter pre-lubricated or in a closed system intermittent catheter bag kit.

The olive-tip catheter can come as a straight or Coude catheter. The difference is that the olive-tip catheter has an olive-shaped looking tip at the end of the catheter. This olive-shaped ball at the tip of the catheter expands a constricted urethra for more natural drainage of urine from the bladder. Along with the straight, Coude catheters, one can also get these catheters in a pre-lubricated sleeve or a closed system intermittent catheter bag kit.

The introducer tip catheter is either a straight or Coude catheter with a protective sleeve that covers the catheter tip until it passes the insertion point of the urethra. The insertion point of the urethra can is a location that can contain a lot of bacteria. The introducer tip protects the catheter tip from getting infected during catheterization, thus protecting the urinary system. The other catheters that are available are the round, the open, the cone, and the whistle tip catheters. These catheters are best suited for specific needs and should be discussed with one's doctor at the rehabilitation center.

The size of all catheters is gauged in the French (FR) scale or French gauge system. The FR number indicates the diameter of the catheter tube. The higher the number, the larger the width of the catheter, 1 FR is equal to 3mm, so a catheter with an FR size of 14 is equal to 4.7mm in diameter.

Catheter lengths vary and should be determined by one's doctor. This decision is based on the patient's body type and the procedure to be carried out. Pediatric catheters are around 10 inches, female catheters are about 6-8 inches (25 cm), and male or unisex catheters are approximately 16 inches (40 and 45 cm) long.

Having the right size diameter catheter is essential. If one can use a catheter with a smaller diameter than what is needed, then emptying the bladder will take time, and there will be leakage of urine. If the catheter diameter is too big, then there will be pain, discomfort, and difficulty inserting the catheter and is more likely to cause trauma to the urethra. The general rule is to select a catheter that is smallest in size without leakage that is suitable to allow adequate drainage. I happen to use a FR 12 straight tip red rubber catheter.

Catheter coatings are essential when choosing a catheter that you will be using daily. Coated intermittent catheters were developed with the intent to help reduce long term complications of the urethra due to daily catheterization (Catheters). One can also purchase intermittent catheters without a coating and apply a gel manually to them. The sterile catheter gel that I use at home daily is called Surgilube. It comes in individual packs or tubes in many different sizes (pictures shown below). Then there are ready to use pre-coated single-use catheters. These catheters have a hydrophilic coating, gel on the catheter surface, or gel inside the catheter packaging. These pre-coated single-use catheters allow for smooth insertion and removal, lowering the chances of irritation. The main two types of pre-coated single-use intermittent catheters are hydrophilic coated catheters and antibiotic coated catheters (Catheters).

- **Hydrophilic coated intermittent catheters:** These coated catheters have a polymer coating, which makes the catheter surface slippery when soaking them in the water or saline right before being used (Catheters).
- **Antibiotic coated intermittent catheters:** The coating on the surface of these catheters produces local antibacterial activity to prevent the risk of a

urinary tract infection (UTI) (Catheters).

When selecting the right coated intermittent catheter, it is best to get a sample package from a medical supplier that has a variety of catheters that they supply. Then try out the multiple intermittent catheters and see which one works the best for you. Below are some pictures of all the different types of catheters, legs bags that I have covered.

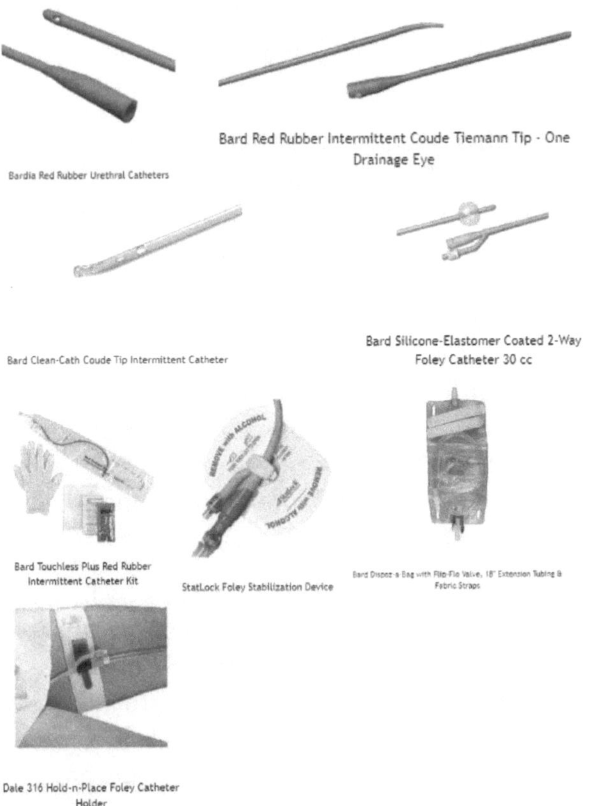

Bardia Red Rubber Urethral Catheters

Bard Red Rubber Intermittent Coude Tiemann Tip - One Drainage Eye

Bard Clean-Cath Coude Tip Intermittent Catheter

Bard Silicone-Elastomer Coated 2-Way Foley Catheter 30 cc

Bard Touchless Plus Red Rubber Intermittent Catheter Kit

StatLock Foley Stabilization Device

Bard Dispoz-a Bag with Flip-Flo Valve, 18" Extension Tubing & Fabric Straps

Dale 316 Hold-n-Place Foley Catheter Holder

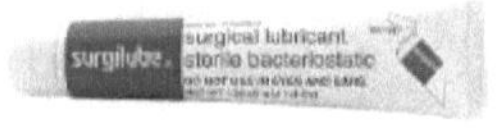

Surgilube Lubricating Jelly - 4.25 oz.
Flip Top Cap

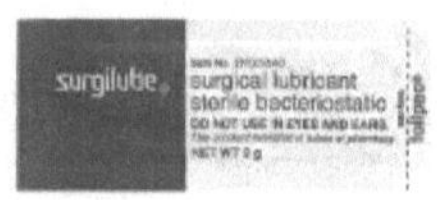

Surgilube Lubricating Jelly 3gm FoilPac

The catheter supplies that I did not cover in this section were the Foley catheter, the condom catheter or external catheter, and the urine leg bag or urostomy pouch. I did not include the Foley catheter or the condom catheters because I do not have any experience in using them.

Other means of cathing are the urine collection leg bag or urostomy pouch since I have used these items in the past and might use it again for long airline flights in the future. The urine collection bag (leg bag) or urostomy pouch is used along with a catheter that has been inserted into the urethra. One may have had to use a catheter and urostomy bag if you have had urinary incontinence (leakage), urinary retention, or surgery. Urinary leg bags come in several different styles to suit personal preference, including disposable and reusable (Vitality).

Choosing a urinary leg bag will be primarily dependent upon one's personal preferences or what one's doctor recommends. Some of the most popular kinds of urinary leg bags include flip valve bags, twist valve bags, stretchable strap leg bags, latex-free leg bags,

reusable leg bags, and disposable leg bags
(Vitality).

- **Flip Valve Bags:** These urinary leg bags have a flip valve that allows quick emptying of the bag and is ideal for oneself that has any issues with a good hand grip (Vitality).
- **Twist Valve Bags:** These urinary leg bags have a twist cap valve to drain quickly, non-hassle emptying, and is an excellent choice for someone that has no issues with a good hand grip (Vitality).
- **Stretchable Strap Leg Bags:** These urinary leg bags with stretchable straps are ideal for people who prefer this type of leg attachment style and can easily be removed by patients with limited hand mobility and strength (Vitality).
- **Latex-free Leg Bags:** These Latex-free urinary leg bags with straps are made from a soft, latex-free material and are ideal for oneself with skin sensitivity or are allergic to latex (Vitality).
- **Reusable Leg Bags:** A reusable urinary leg bag might be the right choice for oneself if you live an active lifestyle and are searching for a urinary leg bag that

provides odor protection (Vitality).

- **Disposable Leg Bags:** A disposable urinary leg bag might be right for oneself if you are searching for a single-use urinary leg bag that can withstand everyday wear and tear, yet disposable (Vitality).

There is a diagram on the next page as to where to attach a urinary leg bag to one's body for natural bladder drainage and accessibility. The leg bags shown in the diagram have an anti-reflux valve, which ensures free-flowing uninterrupted, problem-free usage and built-in odor barrier.

These leg bags will either have a twist or flip valve type drainage port.

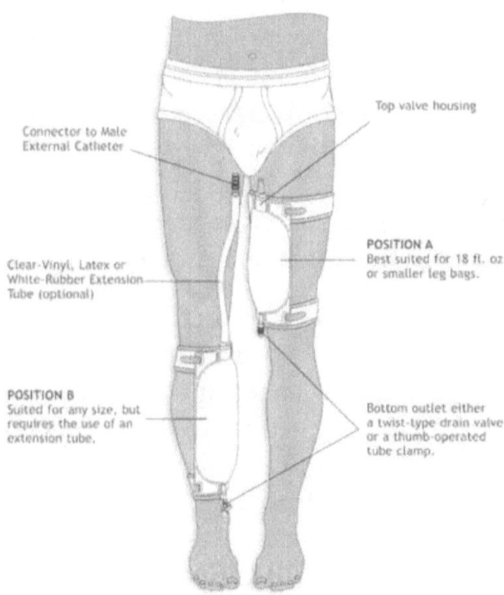

Health and Nutrition

Good health depends on good nutritional foods. Food affects how we look, feel, and how our bodies work (Health). Eating the right foods provide bodies with energy for daily tasks, helps the immune system, and helps maintain proper body weight. Eating a well-balanced diet is essential for people who are paralyzed. As we all know, eating the wrong foods can lead to weight gain, diabetes, heart disease, cancer, joint and muscle injuries, and other ailments (Health).

Due to changes that occur to the body after a SCI, trauma, or disease that causes paralysis, it is more important than ever to understand the role that nutrition plays in maintaining good health. After a person has a spinal cord injury, most people lose some weight due mostly to stress (Health). The injury itself puts stress on the body as it is trying to repair itself. Stress turns up the volume of a person's metabolic rate, which makes the body burn calories much faster than average. As the person's muscles atrophy, the weight loss continues, but only for about a month (Health). The problem after this that most people gain to much weight after their muscles atrophy. People living with a spinal cord injury or paralysis are more prone to inactivity, thus are the reasons for weight gain and even obesity.

There are no clear guidelines on what a person with SCI should or shouldn't eat as part of their balanced diet. The best way for a person with SCI to figure out what works for them is to eat healthy foods, reduce the amount consumed, get some exercise, don't smoke, and do all things in moderation.

When learning what one can and cannot eat after being paralyzed, I would take notes. For example, before my paralysis, I could eat a huge salad or lots of steamed broccoli or steamed cabbage without any digestive issues. Now due to my paralysis causing my body to have a prolonged digestive system, if I overeat these things, my digestive system gives me lots of uncomforting intestinal gas. I have had to learn that I can enjoy these foods but much smaller portions. Until one relearns how the body will react to certain foods. These notes will also come in handy when trying to figure out what is affecting bowel movements.

Bowel Management

Bowel management is directly related to one's diet, the medicines one is taking, and how much water consumed daily. Based on the type of paralysis one is facing, the body might or might not have control of the muscles that control bowel movements. Uncontrollable digestive system muscles make it hard for the body to digest foods. The recommended daily diet would be high in fiber, 20 to 35 grams of fiber each day, and plenty of fluids. Basic regular fiber sources are vegetables, fruits, nuts, popcorn. Also, taking a fiber supplement to help obtain this recommended daily amount. What should be avoided is foods high in fat that don't move through the digestive system very quickly.

When at the rehabilitation center, start to talk to one's nurse or occupational therapist about the bowel movement program. Get an idea as to the best time of day works best for you to complete this program. I do my bowel movement program in the evening, right before I go to bed. But, one might choose to do the bowel movement program early in the morning before breakfast. No matter what time of day one decides to do the bowel movement program, it is always best to do it each day. I would not recommend skipping a day of doing the bowel management program. It is okay not to have a bowel movement each day, but multiple days is not good. If you have no bowel movement for many days in a row, this may be a sign of constipation or bowel blockage.

When living with paralysis, it is vital to understand, know how one's digestive tract functions, and how to manage bowel complications to live a healthy life (Health). Based on the level of one's injury: an injury at or above the L1 result in an upper motor neuron (UMN) bowel syndrome, and if one has an injury below the L1, one has a lower motor neuron (LMN) bowel syndrome. Most people will use either a suppository or a mini-enema to begin their bowel movement program. I used a suppository called the magic bullet for many years, but now this suppository no longer works for me. My body has adjusted, and I no longer need to use a suppository or mini-enema for my bowel movement program, just digital stimulation. One's body will change in this area over time too. The suppository or mini-enema will take approximately 15 to 20 minutes to begin working. After this short waiting period, digital stimulation will need to be performed every 10 to 15 minutes until the rectum is empty. Those with a lower motor neuron (LMN), injury below L1, will typically start their bowel management program with digital stimulation or manual removal (Health). Having an injury below L1 will result in loss of stool movement, slow stool propulsion, which can result in constipation and a higher risk of incontinence (Health). Other risks are hemorrhoids, so use stool softeners, and minimal strain during bowel movements.

Bowel management programs typically last between 30 to 60 minutes to complete. The bowel program is preferably done on the commode. People that are a high risk of skin breakdown should consider doing their bowel program in the lying down position.

Constipation is a problem for people facing paralysis. The daily use of stool softeners or laxatives can help with preventing constipation. Metamucil is a high fiber laxative that can be taken to help move stool through the bowels. Stool softeners like Senna, Docusate, and Colace help keep water contained in the stool, which keeps it softer thus more natural to move. Continued daily use of these stimulants will eventually make the bowels dependent on them.

Healthy Body Weight

Maintaining healthy body weight is vital for a paralyzed person. It is essential not to be overweight as well as underweight. And right now, I have confused you. What I'm telling you is that both can be dangerous to one's health. Being overweight can lead to many health issues ranging from diabetes, heart disease, cancer, and joint and muscle injuries. Being underweight can also lead to health issues ranging from the increased risk for infections, pressure sores, and less energy and fatigue (Health).

Basic nutritional guidelines:

Caloric intake: One's daily balanced caloric intake, it is best to think of low fat, high fiber, and smaller portion sizes. It will take time to figure out. Try to consume only enough food that will allow getting through the day without any hunger cravings. The process of preventing unnecessary weight gain and keep the ideal healthy body weight will take time to learn.

Protein intake: People with a SCI or paralysis generally need more protein in their daily diets. A diet high in protein will help prevent tissue or muscle damage. Eight ounces of high protein should be consumed daily. Eat more protein if developing pressure sore or other skin issues, but don't overdo it. Pay attention to the protein portions, the amount of its fat and cholesterol content. Vitamins that aid in the healing process of the skin are zinc and vitamin C.

Calcium intake: If facing a higher rate of osteoporosis in the lower portion of the body, one should consider adding more vitamin D or calcium-rich foods to the daily diet. Vitamin D helps increase blood circulation and reduce the loss of bone mass. Vitamin D supplements and dairy products with low-fat content are a good source of vitamin D.

Fiber intake: Fiber intake is essential for promoting healthy bowel functioning, preventing constipation, and diarrhea. Nutritionists recommend a daily high fiber diet, which consists of 25-35 grams of whole-grain bread, peanut butter, raw nuts, mixed seeds with dried fruits, cereals, fresh fruits and vegetables, and popcorn. Fiber also prevents diabetes.

Fluid intake: Water is the best fluid to keep hydrated. It helps the digestion system, body temperature, preventing urinary tract infections (UTIs), preventing kidney and bladder stones, and regulates bowel management. Drinking at least eight cups (64 oz.) of water daily is recommended for individuals living with paralysis.

Vitamins and Supplements

Minerals and vitamins: Vitamins A, B, C, and zinc are all good for keeping the skin healthy. Vitamins A and B can be found naturally in fruits and vegetables, whereas good sources for extra zinc and vitamin C can be found in supplement form.

Antioxidant vitamins: If not familiar with antioxidants, they are vitamins like beta-carotene and vitamin C, which inhibits oxidation or reactions promoted by oxygen, peroxides, or free radicals. Antioxidant vitamins attack things inside the body that can damage the body cells and the immune system (Health). Fruits and vegetables are an excellent source for vitamin A (beta-carotene), C, and E.

Vitamin D: An excellent source of vitamin D is sunshine, but if one can get out in it, many supplements are a healthy addition to the daily diet. Other sources of vitamin D are fish-liver oils, egg yolk, and milk.

Pressure Ulcers – Signs of, Preventing and Healing

Pressure ulcers are the leading deadliest injury that a paralyzed person can face in life. About 2.5 million people get pressure ulcers each year. About 60,000 of those people that have a SCI died each year due to getting a pressure ulcer. They are one of the many dangers that a person with a SCI cannot afford to get, have, or even deal with in life. Below I will cover the signs of getting a pressure sore, what are the leading causes of a pressure sore, how to heal a pressure sore, and the danger and life-threatening issues with having a pressure sore. Then I will cover additional health issues that paralyzed people can face and how to prevent them as well.

Pressure ulcers: What is a pressure sore? A pressure ulcer/sore is an injury to the skin and the underlying tissue resulting from constant or continuous pressure on the skin (Mayo). They can develop within hours or days. Pressure ulcers/sores often occur on the skin in the following areas: tailbone or buttock, shoulder blades or spine, back of arms and legs where they rest on the wheelchair (Mayo). The symptoms of pressure sores are:

- Unusual changes to the skin color or texture
- Swelling
- Pus-like draining
- The skin will feel colder or warmer than the surrounding areas
- Tenderness

If one sees any of the above signs of a pressure sore developing, one should change body position or lift body more often per hour. But overall, the best solution is to get out of the wheelchair to relieve total pressure on the affected area. If the skin in this area doesn't show signs of improvement within 24 to 48 hours, contact the doctor. If one's pressure sore has gotten worse, shows signs of infection, have had puss or fluid drainage from the sore, the sore has increased in redness, swelling, warmth, one should seek medical help immediately! Pressure sores are NOT something to take lightly!

The primary causes of pressure sores are:

Pressure: Pressure that is applied continuously to any part of the body can lessen the blood flow, which delivers oxygen, nutrients to the skin tissue. This constant pressure can cause damaged skin to die eventually. The areas of the body that most paralyzed people get pressure sores are the shoulder blades, buttock, spine, hips, and back of the arms and legs where they rest against the wheelchair.

Friction: Friction is the rubbing of the skin against clothing or bedding. If the skin is moist, this friction can cause a pressure sore.

Shear: Shear is a form of friction where the skin is moving in one direction, and the clothing or bedding is moving in another direction. Shear can happen slides or shifts the body across the bed or when slides off the side of the bed onto a wheelchair instead of lifting the body and making an excellent transfer. Shear is mainly caused by not doing proper transfers.

When one has difficulty moving or changing body positions while in bed or while in the wheelchair, the chances increase of getting a pressure sore. Other risk factors that have an impact of getting a pressure sore are immobility, incontinence, lack of skin perception, poor nutrition, and hydration, and any medical condition that affects blood flow.

The complications of a pressure sore that are life-threatening are:

Cellulitis: A common, potentially dangerous bacterial skin infection that can affect paralyzed individuals. It is hazardous for paralyzed individuals because one will not feel its pain.

Bone and Joint Infection: The infection of pressure sore can burrow into the bones and joints. This joint infection is called septic arthritis. It can damage cartilage and tissue. Osteomyelitis is a bone infection that can reduce the functions of joints and limbs (Mayo).

Cancer: Skin cancer cells can develop from long term, non-healing wounds.

Sepsis: Sepsis is a potentially life-threatening condition caused by the body's response to an infection. Sepsis can lead to damage to multiple organ systems in the body.

Prevention of getting a pressure sore all starts with repositioning, shifting the body frequently in the wheelchair, and having a good wheelchair cushion. When it comes to wheelchair cushions, I would recommend getting a Roho Quadtro Select Mid Profile wheelchair cushion.

Here are some additional tips and recommendations for preventing pressure sores:

- I would recommend lifting the body by doing a wheelchair pushup once every 20 to 30 minutes for at least two minutes each time. A wheelchair pushup is done by lifting the body off of the wheelchair cushion. A wheelchair pushup is done by pushing upward on the arms or wheels of the wheelchair.

- If one doesn't have the upper body strength to shift or lift the body or do a wheelchair pushup, don't be afraid to ask someone for help or look into purchasing a specialty wheelchair that can tilt, which will relieve pressure.

- Use a cushion or unique bed mattress to relieve pressure, increase blood flow, and help ensure that the body is well supported. I use a Roho Quadtro Select Mid Profile wheelchair cushion. It has four divided sections that give me excellent posture support, comfort, and pressure relief. It can be purchased through Amazon or online at Walmart.

- Other considerations for preventing pressure sores are:
    - Keeping one's skin clean and dry: Wash skin regularly to limit the skin's exposure to moisture, urine, and stool (Mayo).
    - Protect the skin: Use a moisture barrier skin cream to protect the skin from urine and stool. Change clothing and bedding frequently, if needed.
    - Inspect the skin daily: Look over the body daily for any early warning signs of a pressure sore.

Healing a pressure sore requires drinking lots of fluids (water), vitamins, and a diet high in protein to aid in the healing process. Not only diet is essential, but it is crucial to also remain out of the wheelchair, off the affected area for long periods for it to heal faster or not get worse. (See Chapter 3 – Health and Nutrition – Nutritional Guidelines) When caring for a pressure sore, I would recommend changing the bandage twice a day unless the pressure sore happens to be draining a lot of pus, then I would change the dressing more frequently. If the pressure sore continues to drain pus after four days and also appears not to get any better, I would recommend contacting one's doctor immediately. Pressure sores are NOT something to take lightly!

Infection and Complications

The infection and complications that will be covered in this section are hazardous to people with paralysis. They can lead to life-threatening situations because the symptoms and signs are likely to be missed by a person who is paralyzed. These infections and complications involve the bladder and kidneys. They are preventable!

Urinary tract infection (UTI): Individuals that drink a lot of carbonated beverages (soft drinks), orange juice, and grapefruit juice are more likely to get a UTI. These beverages cause the urine to become alkaline, a breeding ground for bacteria. The best way to prevent UTIs is to wash hands regularly before and after catheterization, use gloves, iodine pads, catheter kits when possible, wipe carefully from front to back, and drink lots of water daily. (See Chapter 3 – Medical Supplies)

Some of the symptoms and signs of a UTI are:

- Blood in urine
- Urine smells bad
- Pain or pressure in the lower back or abdominal area (if one can feel these areas)
- Burning sensation or pain when urinating (one might not be able to feel this)
- Frequent urination, leaking urine and waking up from sleep to urinate (one might not be able to do this)

Kidney or bladder stones: Individuals with SCI may be prone to bladder or kidney stones (Health). One is most likely to get calcium crystals in the urine by drinking sugary beverages like beer, coffee, cocoa, and soft drinks. Eating lots of dairy products like milk, cheese, yogurt, and ice cream can also lead to having kidney or bladder troubles. The best and only way to avoid kidney or bladder stones is to stay hydrated daily by drinking a lot of water.

Kidney Infection: Requires prompt medical attention. If not treated immediately, a kidney infection can permanently damage the kidneys, or the bacteria can spread to the bloodstream, which is a life-threatening situation. Kidney infections are hazardous for people who are paralyzed. Most symptoms and signs of a kidney infection are not noticeable due to paralysis.

The first symptoms and signs of a kidney infection are:

- Fever
- Chills
- Change in color of urine
- Back, side or groin pain (if one can feel these areas)
- Abdominal pain (if one can feel this area)
- Frequent urination (one might not be able to do this)
- Yellowing of the skin (contact one's doctor immediately! – kidneys are shutting down)
- Burning sensation or pain when urinating (one might not be able to feel this)
- Nausea and vomiting
- Pus or blood in the urine
- Urine smells bad or is cloudy

Mental Health – Coping and Adjustment

I know mental health is a very touchy subject, and I am not an expert in mental health by any means. I am discussing mental health because it affected me personally when dealing with my struggle of being paralyzed. I want to help people, so, therefore, I am willing to talk about it. I went through hard times while facing my paralysis, all the feelings about being paralyzed, all while learning to adapt to my new life. You are NOT alone! There were about two weeks that I struggled to even think about getting out of bed or also get up to get something to eat, brush my teeth, or take a shower. I think most of the people that face adapting their life to being paralyzed will have to meet all sorts of negative feelings like loss, denial, helplessness, regret, why-me, second-guessing, depression, doubt, sadness and uncertainty.

In the beginning, many people react to paralysis like there is nothing wrong or nothing happened. They don't want to accept the changes to their body or why they can't move. Some may even see their paralysis as an annoyance as I did for my first couple of days in rehabilitation. It's okay to be in denial, and I was at first, too. Denial is just part of the healing process to get through the shocking news of being paralyzed. In the denial stage of healing, people will either become inactive, do nothing or do too much, try to overcome, and compensate for the physical limitations. Don't use this denial stage to keep one from enjoying life, getting motivated, or pushing oneself. Overcome it and be focused on adapting to one's new life. Adapt, overcome, and be strong!

When the denial is gone, most people will replace the denial with anger, rage, and resentment. I also went through this part of the healing process. Anger is not very healthy and hinders the healing process. It is another defense mechanism to becoming paralyzed. Being frustrated, lashing out at the people who are trying to help oneself is also part of this stage of healing. I know that this will be hard, but try not to be this way, hurting the people that are trying to help themselves during this challenging stage in one's life. Being hurtful to others that care about you is not productive in one's overall healing process. You do not want to say anything that one will regret later or can take back through apologizing.

Fear and extreme sadness are other feelings that are common after paralysis. The fear of losing control of one's life as it was, facing a new life in a wheelchair, and fear of the unknown are some of the many feelings that one will encounter while adapting to being paralyzed. Sadness passes. When someone faces grief or also called the blues, this will pass. I faced a time of sadness, as well. I used all the positive things in my life, like family, friends, and my dog to help me pull through this phase. It's important not to confuse sadness, blues with the medical condition depression. Depression can lead to a range of issues like difficulty concentrating, inactivity, and feelings of hopelessness, worthlessness, and drastic change in appetite or sleep time. A person facing depression may have thoughts about suicide. Suicide affects people with SCI more than non-disabled people. Suicide is the leading cause of death for people younger than 55 that have a spinal cord injury (Health). If you or someone you love shows any signs of depression, I would immediately seek professional help. Depression is not something one or a loved one should face alone.

Do not let all the negative feelings affect one's health. I know that this is much easier said than done. The last thing one wants to face is a health issue that is in addition to being paralyzed. When facing paralysis, a person's feelings might also affect the way they take care of their bladder or skin or nutrition. People that have a history of alcohol or substance abuse may return to their old patterns of self-destruction to quiet their anxieties or fears/feelings (Health). During this time of facing all sorts of emotions, trying to rebuild one's life back to where it was before paralysis, people sometimes start to neglect their care. Health problems one may face during this time of negativity could be urinary tract infections, respiratory complications, and pressure sores. This time of negativity is the time to reach out to family, friends, and peer groups in one's community. Talk to people close to you or people that can relate to one's paralysis about anything that's on one's mind or affecting one's personal feelings, health issues. It is also a great time to ask people for help in anything that one needs to be done that one cannot complete, things like doing the laundry, making the bed, vacuuming the floors, cleaning the bathroom, changing a light bulb, and more. Don't be afraid to ask for help!

What helped me the most to get through all the negative thoughts and feelings while facing my paralysis was to reach out to anyone that would listen. I reached out to my family, my friends, and just about basically anyone that I could just talk to and connect with, even total strangers at my rehabilitation center. I researched on the internet my type of paralysis, health issues that people face when paralyzed, new technology being studied and used to help paralyzed people walk again, how to cope with paralysis, peer groups that were available to talk to about the issues. Using the internet during this time for me was very helpful, a valuable tool, and I learned a lot about how to cope, live with paralysis. I also learned that just talking about issues I was facing helped me become more robust, have hope, focus on becoming a better person, and get through this drastic change in my life. Knowing that I had family, friends that were just a phone call away that were willing to help me get through these hard times was also helpful for me. If one doesn't have family or friends that are close by, I would suggest that you reach out to someone that is facing a similar paralysis. Reaching out to someone with the same paralysis will help one to relate to them, make a new friend, be able to talk freely about all the issues that you both have been facing. Also, one can search for peer groups at the local rehabilitation centers. Most rehabilitation centers have weekly peer groups that meet to talk about all the issues that people are facing in their new life after being paralyzed. You are NOT alone! Many people suffer from depression, emotions of uncertainty after being paralyzed. I know that this sounds simple, but all one must do is reach out to loved ones, family, friends, and peer groups, and they will be there for you for emotional and physical support through this hard time in one's life. You will get through this!

If there are no peer groups, family and friends are not available. I would suggest finding something constructive that will help one occupy one's mind and time. Here are some ideas that I had thought about doing to keep myself from becoming depressed: writing an e-book, building model cars or airplanes, designing a website, designing a new wheelchair, researching adaptive sports in the area, and taking some online college courses. I also used this time to relearn how to get fully dressed, cook some meals by myself, and make better transfers to different pieces of furniture. I know it is easy to talk about depression, sadness, doubt, but I know from experience that you can beat this. Just keep one's mind busy, time, and the depressive state will past. I pulled through my depression state with flying colors, and you can too. I believe in YOU!

With time one will reach the final stage of the grieving process, accept the realistic view of one's paralysis, and start making plans for one's new life ahead. Adjustment to one's new life will depend on self-motivation. When I was focusing on starting my new life, I focused first on my physical strength. (I will cover more about exercise programs later in chapter four) Physical strength is what one will have to depend on daily for pushing the wheelchair and for transferring. I then focused on my personal goals of finishing college, getting a good job, and getting married. Don't get me wrong; all this time, I was still hoping to regain my ability to walk again. Hope is excellent, not unrealistic, but don't stop moving forward on one's own life goals to wait for a cure, this is a sign of denial. Get motivated, strong-willed, and focus on one's personal goals and the good things in life!

I know that getting things done after paralysis is a significant challenge, will take more time than average to complete a simple task like getting dressed. I have been there; I know some of the many challenges one will face. I had to relearn how to get dressed, move around the house, cook meals, and more. Don't be ashamed to ask for help; asking for help is okay. It's how one may be able to get things done. Adjustment to paralysis is a daily process, will take time to change one's thoughts, feelings, and behavior. It takes time to rebuild one's life, identity, and find balance in life (Health). Face every challenge head-on, find or figure out solutions to every challenge that one will face daily. Facing these daily challenges will make a stronger you, a better person, and give oneself motivation and hope. I believe in YOU!

Chapter 4

Don't Panic! You WILL fall!

We are going to talk about when one falls out of the wheelchair. Falls from a wheelchair are emanated; being prepared is very important. Did one cover the many ways on how to get back into the wheelchair while at the rehabilitation center? If you did, this is great! I learned many techniques on how to recover from falling out of my wheelchair at my rehabilitation center, but I honed my technique after I returned home and discovered the best way for myself. I have fallen out of my wheelchair I think three times in five years which is not too bad. Two of the times that I have fallen out of my wheelchair were when I wouldn't even have thought that I would have fallen. One time, I was doing a regular transfer that I had done many, many times before. I just didn't raise my lower body high enough to make the proper transfer, and then I ended up on the floor between my wheelchair and my bed. The other time, I ended up on the floor between my wheelchair and the living room couch. Oh, and the third time was between the bathroom toilet, the tub, which wasn't the most pleasant fall of them all since I had just finished my bathroom program. I was in the process of heading off to bed for the night, and luckily my brother was there to help me get back into my wheelchair. There are three possible main reasons why one will fall when you at least expect it to happen. In the first scenario, one will not make an excellent proper transfer, and before one knows it, it's too late, you are on the floor. The second scenario is when one's arms or upper body are fatigued from daily tasks. When one goes to make a transfer, the body just will not cooperate, which then puts you on the floor. The third possible scenario is to fall when one thinks that they won't fall. Then it happens, and one has no clue as to why or how one ended up on the floor.

Now, by not knowing when one will fall out of the wheelchair, it is hard to prepare oneself for this when it happens. My first words of advice are DO NOT PANIC! Compose oneself! Make sure that you're not injured, then look around to see what objects are solid enough to be used to push oneself back up into the wheelchair. If there is no one about to help, take one's time pushing oneself back up into the wheelchair. Since one doesn't push oneself up from the floor level often, this will be a slight challenge. It might take more than one attempt to lift oneself back into the wheelchair.

My first time falling, it took me three attempts before I could get myself firmly seated back into my wheelchair. If there is someone around when one falls, don't feel too embarrassed to ask them for help politely. We all have bad days, even people that are not paralyzed and in wheelchairs fall. Brush oneself off, learn from it, and get on with life. Now, when one does ask someone for help, try to instruct the person helping you on the proper way to lifting one's body back into the wheelchair. You don't want them to drop you and cause an injury while trying to help. If a person offers to help, advise them to hook their arms under one's armpits and lift upward as oneself is also pressing upward on a stable, immovable object or the front of the wheelchair frame until firmly seated back onto the wheelchair cushion. If there is no one around to help, the first step is to see what is around that is anchored and will not move when applying all of one's body weight onto it, to push oneself back up onto the wheelchair. If there is a couch nearby, to make things easier, remove one of the cushions from the sofa. Then place one's body between the wheelchair and the sofa. Then lock the brakes on the wheelchair, use the front frame of the wheelchair to push oneself up onto the couch where the cushion has been removed. Then shift one's body over onto one of the couch cushions so that you're now higher than before. At this point, one should be able to transfer back into the wheelchair. Take one's time! You do not want to make all this effort and work just to end up back on the floor again. So, again, you will fall, just DO NOT PANIC!

Exercise and Preventing Injury

In this section, we will cover the importance of exercise for people that use manual wheelchairs, how to prevent muscle, joint injury, and the extreme importance of checking one's skin daily. People that use a manual wheelchair daily must depend on their hands, wrists, arms, shoulders, chest, and upper back muscles for their daily routine. It is essential to have a daily routine that involves any physical activity that helps keep the bodyweight manageable and one's upper body strength to a level that makes mobility easier in life. A paralyzed person depends daily on their upper body strength for movement, transfers, and daily routine. So, it is vital to keep this part of the body healthy and without injury. If one sustains an injury to the upper body muscles and or joints, this would mean that one is down for the count. One's daily routine would be no more until healed. Therefore, it is essential to have some form of regular exercise routine along with healthy activities to maintain or reduce body weight and to build the necessary muscles that one needs to live healthily.

Bodyweight is one of the leading causes of muscle or joint injury for a person that uses a manual wheelchair and can also contribute to getting a pressure sore. If the body gets too heavy, then this adds more stress and pressure on the muscles and joints during daily activities, which can lead to an injury or even worse surgery. So, again, I cannot express more the importance of a regular exercise routine!

The most common injury for manual wheelchair users is a shoulder injury. The shoulder is a vital joint and muscle group that is used daily in performing transfers, pressure relief, and basic movements in one's wheelchair. The first step to preventing and avoiding a shoulder injury is having the right wheelchair for you. (See Chapter 2 – Adaptability and Mobility Equipment) A full-time manual wheelchair user should use a fully customizable wheelchair made of the lightest possible materials. This manual wheelchair should be configured and adjusted to fit one's body like a glove. The most important adjustment that needs to be made is the axle position. Axle position provides the smoothest roll, least resistance, increases one's efficiency of a push, and minimizes the risk of a shoulder injury.

You will know that the wheelchair's axle is in the correct position when one reaches down to one's side, and the middle finger is pointing to the shaft. When setting up one's manual wheelchair for the first time, it is best to seek the help of a wheelchair or seating therapist. When purchasing a customizable manual wheelchair, always keep in mind the weight of each component that you add to the chair. The fully customizable manual wheelchair base weight might start at 15 pounds, but by the time you add the weight of the cushion, the wheels, the casters, and the chair back. One's fully customizable wheelchair total weight might end being up to closer to 22 pounds. The weight one will be pushing plus body weight each time one pushes. So, think about all this weight being applied to one's shoulders and how it affects other parts of one's arms during each push.

Preventing a shoulder injury starts with the right equipment, which we covered above.

Now, let's talk about back posture and daily stretching. These two things can also prevent a shoulder injury. Bad or slumped posture starts with sitting in a wheelchair all day. Slumped posture leads to longer back muscles and shorter stomach muscles. The lousy posture and shorter stomach muscles lead to decreased shoulder range of motion, inefficient push, and shoulder pain or injury. Daily stretching is essential! With the right equipment and good posture, it is possible to push a manual wheelchair one's entire life without shoulder pain or injury or surgery. The many factors that will begin to make it more challenging to drive a manual wheelchair day to day are living where there is rough terrain or hills, age, body weight, or prior injury or pain. When this time comes, one will have to decide to start using a power assist device or change to using a specialty motorized wheelchair.

Let's start by talking about a new exercise program. I would consider thinking about the following questions before starting. Should you work with an exercise trainer for a while before working out on one's own? How much weight will one be lifting (weightlifting) while seated in the wheelchair? What is the maximum amount of weight that one's wheelchair can hold? (One's body weight plus the total amount of weight that one will be lifting) Will one be using free weights or cable weight machines for one's exercises? Consider what impact the exercise program will have on one's skin. Make sure that you are considering this as well, add padding under one's body where needed to perform any exercise. You do not want to end up getting a pressure sore due to you trying to get into shape or loss bodyweight. After you have considered all these questions, issues regarding performing a new exercise routine, then I would change and adapt one's exercise plan according to these answers. If you have never done an exercise program or think that you will need help getting one started, please do not hesitate to consult with a personal exercise trainer at a gym or rehabilitation center near where you live. These people are here to help. They can show you proper lifting form, create an exercise program based on one's needs, abilities, and goals. All of these things will get you started in the right direction towards a healthy exercise program.

When performing each exercise, think about the safety of one's muscles and joints. To prevent possible injury during the exercise program, in the future, start the exercise program with a warmup period. This warmup period needs to last at least 15 to 20 minutes and should include all the muscles that one is planning on working out that day. And remember, it is best to prevent muscle injury by starting the exercise routine with lightweight first, then slowly move up to heavier weight as you progress. Also, concentrate on one's form while performing the exercise and not on how much weight being lifted. Correct body form, the use of moderate weight while performing a task will lessen the chances of injury during the exercise program.

During the exercise program, remember to take some short breaks to keep hydrated by drinking lots of water, when possible checking one's skin for signs of tenderness or the beginning of a pressure sore, ulcer. A pressure sore can happen at any time when the skin is not tough enough, too much pressure, body heat is applied to a small area of skin. It is best to start with small amounts of time doing one's exercise program, then slowly increase the amount of time like increasing the amount of weight one is using. This slow increase in time performing one's exercise program will give the skin the time it needs to get tougher; this time will help prevent the skin from turning into a pressure sore very fast. I would start by seeing how much of the exercise program that one can complete in 15 minutes. Then increase this time every five days by 15 minutes, while checking one's skin daily for any signs of the surface being tender or an abrasion. If signs of a pressure sore start to appear, skin becoming tender take time off from the exercise program for a few days to see if the skin recovers and becomes normal again. If the skin recovers, then continue the exercise program. If the skin doesn't recover, give it more time to do this. Think of it this way, the healthier one's skin remains, the more one can work out, get into shape, and become more robust too. One does not want an ulcer/pressure sore when just starting to get going on working out program, and this would be a lot to handle, can set one back on getting to enjoy all the things that one wants to do in life. Take this advice from a very active guy who pushed himself, didn't slow down, and take care of his skin as he should have. Then ended up fighting a pressure sore for over a year, and ended up having flap surgery in the end. So, I urge you to please take good care of one's skin!

All of the following things that will prevent a pressure sore and a possible shoulder injury: good care of one's skin (no pressure sores), having a daily exercise program to keep one's bodyweight manageable, keeping upper body strength to a level that makes mobility easier, eating healthy, a correct setup wheelchair. Shoulder surgery or replacement is NOT something you want to experience. So, again, I cannot express the importance of a daily exercise program!

Playing Adaptive Sports

In this section, we are going to cover playing adaptive sports. There are a lot of adaptive sports available to play. All one must do is research what sports are available in the area, connect with the contact person(s) through the sport's Facebook page, or the sport's website, and get started. Here is a list of adaptable sports in my city, Charlotte, NC: sled hockey, tennis, basketball, water skiing, snow skiing, hand cycling, mountain biking, rock and tree climbing, rugby, curling, kayaking, sailing, scuba diving, and swimming. Pictures of some of the many adaptive sports available here in the United States are shown in the appendix. Many larger cities like New York, NY, Chicago, IL, Los Angeles, CA, Dallas,

TX, and Atlanta, GA, may have a much more extensive selection of adaptive sports available. Do some research, find a sport that one would like to try and possibly enjoy, connect with people, and have some fun!

When you finally connect with the contact person for an adaptive sport that you want to try, make sure that you ask them a lot of questions. Ask the contact person(s) and oneself the following questions: What type of equipment is needed to play the sport? What kind of equipment is necessary for my physical ability to play the sport? How will the body be positioned while playing the sport? Will one be seated in adaptive equipment for the sport? Will one need a specialized cushion for the adaptive equipment? Will the body be shifting around a lot while in a seated position? What other safety or adaptive equipment will one need? (Sled hockey, rugby, snow skiing)

My first adaptive sport, sled hockey, right from the start after I sat down in a sled for the very first time, I was hooked. I had reached out to the contact person, Jereme Gilbert at Queen City Sled Hockey through Facebook. Jereme had been paralyzed about a year or two earlier than me, and he was trying to start a sled hockey team in the Charlotte, NC area. I could relate to Jereme immediately. He was younger than me, but very active, loved playing sports and a great sled hockey coach. I was so eager to get involved, not only learning this new and exciting sport but to help Jereme build a team that I got my first sport-related pressure sore within a few months of playing. I then had to take a month off from playing and let my body heal.

Jereme had already faced a pressure sore, flap surgery by this time in his life, so he knew how imperative it was for me to take this time off from playing very seriously. I healed up, was back on the ice in no time. Jereme and I went on to travel to many cities, playing in many games, tournaments for the following year with the Raleigh, NC Hurricanes sled hockey team. This time-traveling, playing, meeting wonderful people in the sport was so thrilling, very, very exciting for me. Then my life came to an extreme full stop. I had been balancing going to college, working fulltime, playing sled hockey when possible, then I got another pressure sore. This pressure sore would last a full year, end up making me have flap surgery. This time way, from going to college, spending time with friends, playing the new adaptive sport that I came to love, just crushed me. At the time that I am writing this e-book, I am in recovery from having my flap surgery. I must now slowly build up the amount of time that I can be in my chair, let my skin toughen back up, this takes over six months. And after this time passes, then maybe, I can try to get back in the sled to play the excellent sport of sled hockey that I have dearly missed for close to two years now. I can't stress the importance of skincare when playing or learning to play an adaptive sport. So, please hear my concern, warning about taking excellent care of one's skin! Don't go out there and think that getting a pressure sore will never happen to you because that's when it will happen! I don't want you to miss out on spending time with new friends, learning a new adaptive sport.

Chapter 5

Social Meetings and Relationships

As one slowly starts to get one's life back, social meetings, relationships are essential to rekindle and rebuild. Start slow, think about the amount of time that one will be in the wheelchair, think about places that one can go to meet one's friends. Some questions and concerns that one might need to consider before one's first social meeting in public are: Is the meeting places accessible? Are the tables at the meeting place accessible, the height of the tables? Will one be able to move around at the meeting place, enough floor space? How much pushing one will be doing during this time? Will one need to use the bathroom before going out, or do you plan on using the facilities while out? What supplies will one need to take with you? How does the body react to certain foods in case one plan on getting something to eat while out? Knowing what one can and cannot eat will prevent a bowel movement accident in a public place and the embarrassment that follows. And lastly, being out too late, how will this affect one's bowel management program?

Now that one has had a chance to think about all these questions, we can move on to how you will handle one's friend's reactions towards seeing oneself out in public in the wheelchair for the first time. One's friends might look at oneself a little differently, but reassure them that you are the same person as you were before one's paralysis, just a little shorter. One must see the humor in this and smile. I'm a guy that was 5' 10" tall, now a little over 4' tall in my chair. And, yes, one's friends might crack some short jokes about you now. So, just be prepared. Enjoy the moment of going out to spend time with friends or family. Some of my first social outings were with my family. I wanted to feel comfortable in my chair for the first few times, so I chose to go out with my family for a meal at a restaurant. I wanted to see how I would feel about being in public, how I could navigate the restaurant's floor plan, then experience a full meal in society as well. Going out with my family first helped me build my confidence, self-esteem, the experience of eating out, and being in public. I faced many different feelings when going out in society the first few times by myself, but by going out with my family beforehand helped me overcome these feelings and once again enjoy my freedom.

For me, along with regaining my freedom of being able to get out, spend time with my friends, I also expanded my freedom by learning how to drive my vehicle with hand controls. Learning to drive again with hand controls could be a future goal for oneself as well. Being able to drive oneself to visit with friends, family, and even to doctor's appointments is a very nice feeling of the freedom one had missed, that you now desire in one's new life. I would recommend doing some research on the internet about possible hand controls that will work for one's needs, a vehicle that one can safely get in and out of, and a driving school nearby if required by one's state law to take a driving course with the new hand controls. My state of North Carolina requires one to take a driving course using hand controls to get a certificate of completion for the renewal of one's driver's license. Drive safely!

The next topic I would like to cover is about relationships, dating, and marriage to be precise. I was very hesitant to get back out in the dating scene after my paralysis. It took me many times to go out with friends to even remotely feel comfortable about approaching and striking up a conversation with a woman. I know that being in a wheelchair makes it even harder to approach, talk, and even date someone. These are feelings of doubt, lack of self-confidence, but with practice and time, these feelings will pass after many unsuccessful attempts of meeting that special someone in a bar or night club. I decided to skip the bar, club scene, and look towards online dating. After a little over a year of online dating, I was able to meet that extraordinary woman, marry her, and start a new chapter in my life. The lack of my physical abilities didn't stop her from seeing the real person that I am and fall in love with me. I believe that there is someone special out there for all of us. I believe in you!

Chapter 6

Choosing and Starting a New Career

The day finally came for me to get back into the career world. It had been over four years since being paralyzed, not having held a full-time job. At this point in my life, I was able to drive my vehicle with hand controls, maintain a healthy lifestyle, and start to think about a career. When getting back into the career world, one must take into consideration the following questions: Will one be able to perform all the job's physical requirements? The amount of time (travel time) that one will be in the wheelchair? How often will one have to use the facilities? How to plan for a bowel accident? What things (supplies) one will need to take with you to the job? Is this job a full-time or part-time job? Will this employer have to make any special adaptions to desks or workstations for oneself to be able to do the job? Is there handicap access to the building? Is there an elevator in the building? I may have missed some questions, but one can get the picture as to what to think about when taking and starting a new career.

After you have considered all the above questions, one can now focus on any questions or concerns that I may have missed, what type of job to apply for, take, and enjoy. I was in the law enforcement field before my paralysis. I made a career change to information technology. This career change was best suited for me for physical reasons but also because I enjoy learning and working with computers. When applying for a job, take into consideration the physical requirements needed to perform the job. If one thinks you can fulfill all the physical obligations of the job posting, then apply for the job. I have applied for a job that I thought I could perform all the physical requirements. Then I get to the interview part to realize later that I'm not physically able to achieve. Make sure that one can perform the job before applying to it and not waste time. So, read all the job descriptions before questioning whether one can or cannot meet the physical requirements of a job posting. It took me a while to find a job that I could fit all the needs, which is why I chose to make a career change to information technology. It seemed to me to be the right choice for a person limited by reach, lifting ability, and in a wheelchair. I hope that one can find a new career that will build up one's self-esteem, confidence, give one back much satisfaction in life.

After one has accepted a job offer, but before the first day of getting back into the career world, the most important thing is to make a plan, prepare oneself from unforeseen health-related problems. Be prepared. If one thinks, plans about how one would be able to react to an accidental bowel movement or any other health-related issue while at work, one will be able to keep the embarrassment level to a minimum when they do happen. When I first started back to work, I carried in my chair backpack a new brief, at least three catheter kits, a pack of baby wipes, two plastic grocery bags, and extra pair of dress pants and shirts. The plastic grocery bags were for soiled clothes and other types of garbage. My backpack was my daily emergency, anti-embarrassment work kit. Fortunately, I never had to use this emergency cleanup kit, have continued to have good everyday working experience. I hope that one will never have to face an embarrassing situation while at work. Again, it's best to be prepared just in case. Suppose later one feels safe about not having to carry such a large cleanup kit with you to work each day. One can then adjust it to one's daily needs. After being more comfortable, confident about my body, I ended up reducing my everyday kit to just a pack of baby wipes and three catheter kits.

I wish you all the very best wishes in getting back into the career world. Having a career is a huge step towards independence, freedom, more positive self-esteem, more substantial confidence, enjoyment, and satisfaction in life.

Chapter 7

Travel

Yes! Traveling is still very much possible being while paralyzed. Don't let one's paralysis or the wheelchair prevent you from exploring one's state, country, and world. The freedom of traveling is a beautiful life experience, and one shouldn't let being in a wheelchair prevent this. Whether traveling by car, train, or airplane, the experience of traveling is one that you will never forget. Traveling by car, train, or plane is truly a great sign of how far one has come to regaining one's freedom. It is a beautiful feeling to have freedom back in one's life. The first time that I got behind the wheel of my vehicle after my paralysis drove myself to meet some friends for lunch was so exhilarating and exciting. This event put the biggest smile on my face, and nothing could ruin my day from that moment forward. The same feeling for me was when my friend, Jereme, and I took my first plane trip to a sled hockey tournament in Tampa, FL.

I was very excited about the trip, but I also very nervous about my chair being mishandled or damaged or if I would have a health issue during the journey. In the end, I was nervous and worried about nothing. It was the best trip ever after my paralysis, the freedom of traveling, learning a new sport, and making new friends. From this moment forward, Jereme and I continued to trip to many more sled hockey tournaments together. We have flown together to Chicago, Illinois and Tampa, Florida. I have as well driven from Charlotte, North Carolina to Raleigh, North Carolina, and then from Charlotte, North Carolina to Knoxville, Tennessee for sled hockey tournaments. These trips by car were, on average, a little over four hours long.

What I am going to cover in this section is how to prepare oneself when traveling by car or airplane. The best travel plan is to have a plan, and the best philosophy when traveling is to hope for the best but plan for the worst. Planning is essential for people who use adaptive equipment. No plan is one hundred percent bulletproof, especially when it comes to transportation, lodging, scheduling, weather, and all the unforeseen problems that may occur during one's travel (Reeves Foundation). When I plan my trips, I use this helpful, informative website, https://wheelchairjimmy.com/, for all the accessibility questions that I have about the city that I am traveling too. The wheelchair Jimmy website has always been my first stop for information about the cities accessibility. Jim Parsons is the owner of this website and a significant advocate for all wheelchair users when it comes to airline travel. Check out the website's WJAR Ratings, Featured Locations, Advocacy Blog, QuickView Guides, travel tips, and other great features.

For those who have little or no experience with traveling with a wheelchair or any other equipment for one's paralysis, it's a good idea to reach out for the help of someone with a lot of personal experience or a travel agent who specializes in the disability travel market. There are travel agents that know how to get oneself safely where you want to go (Reeves Foundation). I had never used a travel agent but instead reached out to my friend, Jereme, because he had already made many trips before and knew how to prepare for one. Jereme has a similar paralysis as me, and we can relate to each other's needs when traveling together. It is also best to make one's first trip to a destination that is knowledgeable with people with disabilities (Reeves Foundation). My first trip was an airplane ride to a sled hockey tournament in Tampa, Florida. The local hotels where most of the sled hockey players stayed were very accommodating to people with disabilities. The hotel, the ice rink, restaurants were within rolling distance away, which made the trip more enjoyable and much less frustrating. When thinking about planning a trip, think of it in these three stages: getting ready, getting there, and being there.

The getting ready stage of planning one's trip starts with making all the travel arrangements. Start by thinking about what phone calls that one will be needed to make before starting the journey. Thinking about how many days one will need to pack, what medical supplies one will need to take with you, and making sure that you have emergency phone numbers and health insurance information readily available during one's trip. These are just a few things to consider when planning a trip.

Getting there stage of one's trip is all about how one will be traveling to the destination, traveling while at one's destination, and then returning home.

If traveling by vehicle, one will need to think about where the stopping points along one's travel route are for food, gas, bathroom availability, and how one will be lifting the body to prevent a pressure sore. One will also need to think about who will be driving. Will one be doing the driving, or will a friend or family member? If you are not doing the driving, make sure that the person doing the driving knows the stopping point along the route for food, bathroom breaks, and knows one's emergency contact information. It is always best that both you and this person know what to do in case of an emergency. Most travel destinations will have handicap parking, but just to make sure to contact the hotel or travel destination in advance to verify this information.

When traveling by airplane, one will have to do a lot more preparation in advance for the trip. One will need to think about the travel plans to the local airport, the airplane ride, and the travel plan for when one arrives at the destination. Then the plan on how to get one's luggage from the airport to the hotel, the travel plan for going places while at the destination, the travel plan for returning to the airport to fly home. Then the travel plan for getting the luggage from the local airport back to one's home. And these are just the questions that one will need to think about just for traveling. (See the appendix for some additional helpful travel and awesome travel gear websites.)

Here are some additional helpful questions and statements to get started on traveling by airplane:

- How will one travel to the airport?
- How will one travel from the airport to the hotel?
- How will one travel from the hotel to another destination?
- How will one travel from the hotel back to the airport at the end of the trip?
- How will one travel from the airport back to one's home at the end of the trip?
- How many days of medical supplies will one need to pack?
- Will one need to purchase a giant suitcase to carry all one's medical supplies and clothing?
- How will one get the luggage and oneself into and back out of the airport safely?
- Try to book a direct flight when traveling by airplane
- Call the airport the day before the flight to schedule an aisle chair so that they are aware of one's

travel needs (do this for both one's leaving and returning flights)

- When traveling by airplane, make sure there is nothing loose on the wheelchair that could be torn off or damaged
- Take the seat cushion onto the airplane (a Roho or inflated cushion can explode while in the airplane's cargo compartment)
- Use the facilities before boarding a flight, limit liquid intake while in flight, this will prevent unforeseen future health issues
- Lift the body frequently when traveling by car or airplane to prevent a pressure sore
- Pack a backpack for a carry-on bag for all catheter supplies and medicines (Never pack them in the checked luggage) this bag can be used later for a daypack to hold water, clothing, and souvenirs, etc.
- Assume that anyone wearing an airline uniform doesn't know how to help you or handle a wheelchair
- Bring a portable set of Allen wrenches for brake, caster adjustment

- Check the tire air pressure before leaving, pack a portable air pump (Solid rubber wheels are the best option for traveling)
- Boost the immune system by taking a multivitamin or vitamin booster before the trip. Hand sanitizer is helpful, too.
- Compression socks are suitable for circulation and for preventing leg swelling; helps the body stay warm in cold weather
- Medical supplies – always pack more than one will need because you never know – flights get delayed, cars break down, wicked weather brews
- When flying - check-in at the desk instead of the kiosk to arrange for boarding and on-flight wheelchairs, then gate-check one's wheelchair, remove everything that can fall off the wheelchair like side-guards, seat cushions, etc. (Reeves Foundation)
- Protect one's hands! Gloves are an excellent idea to protect one's hands along the sometimes bumpy, dirty road (Reeves Foundation).

- When booking any type of reservation, a plane flight, train ride, hotel, restaurant, etc., one should notify the other party in advance that you are in a wheelchair (Reeves Foundation).
- Enjoy the food on the trip, but don't shock one's stomach! Let the digestive system adjust to new foods and spices. If one doesn't do this, it could lead to indigestion and an irregular bowel (Reeves Foundation).
- When it comes to public restrooms, this sometimes can be very challenging. Try locating a shopping center, chain coffee shops, hotel lobbies, train/subway stations, airports, government buildings, banks, and fast-food restaurants (Reeves Foundation).
- Prepare one's mind, be open to new things that come one's way, whether cuisine or access features, but also when situations don't go according to plan. Go with the flow, and you'll be guaranteed to have a more pleasant and eye-opening experience (Reeves Foundation).

The last stage of planning the trip is the being there stage. When one is planning the trip or while on one's journey, try to keep an open mind that one will not be able to prevent unforeseen events and issues. Be mentally prepared that both positive and negative things will happen during the trip. A negative thought might be getting a flat tire, or the luggage gets lost by the airline. A positive thing might be getting an accessible hotel room with a king-size bed instead of a queen-size bed, or meeting and making new friends on one's trip. Accept all challenges, be open-minded to adapting and changing things that will happen on the trip. Most importantly, enjoy the journey; it's an exciting life experience and an adventure!

Chapter 8

Clinical Research (Stem cells)

In keeping my hopes, dreams alive, I research weekly the advances of treating paralysis with the use of stem cells. An unknown fact about spinal cord injury patients is that 99% who are paralyzed never walk again, so researchers have been focusing on transplanting new cells into the cavity formed by the injured area in the spinal cord. They hope that stem cell therapy will reduce the inflammation that causes further paralysis.

The most promising clinical trials and studies lately involving stem cells are coming from the University of Texas Southwestern Medical Center located in Dallas, Texas, the Mayo Clinic in Rochester, Minnesota, the Keck School of Medicine of the University of Southern California, and the Miami Project to Cure Paralysis. One can also search the website: https://clinicaltrials.gov/ for future clinical trials and studies as they come available throughout the world.

The stem cells that are showing promising effects are called induced pluripotent cells (iPS) and Q stem cells. In 2006, scientists discovered how to "reprogram" cells with a specialized function, and these cells were then induced pluripotent cells (iPS). These cells can become cells of an organ, tissue, and suitable for therapies related to SCI. Q stem cells are cells that have been engineered to repair the central nervous system. These cells, called progenitor cells, scientists are currently studying to be used to improve paralysis. The study of these two types of cells shows there is hope that science will pave the way for repairing the damages of a SCI in the future.

Chapter 9

New Technology and Exoskeleton Suits

The new technology in the area of using computer chips, advancements in the development and design of exoskeleton suits for paralyzed people are constantly changing these days. When I first started to research companies that were building an exoskeleton suit for paralyzed people back in 2014, there were only three that were known. Today, more than twenty companies are researching, developing these advanced exoskeletal suits for paralyzed people. Two of these will know companies are Ekso Bionics located in Berkeley, California, and ReWalk situated in Israel.

Esko Bionics, founded in 2005, continues today to lead the way in the field of exoskeletons, designing and creating some of the most innovative solutions in helping people with mobility and capability issues. Esko Bionics has forged lasting partnerships with the Department of Defense and the Lockheed Martin Corporation.

ReWalk, an Israeli start-up in 2014, received FDA approval, clearance for rehabilitation use in the United States. Their exoskeleton suit is designed to aid movement for people with lower-body paralysis. The ReWalk wearable robotic exoskeleton suit provides power to hip, knee motion. This suit enables paralyzed individuals with a SCI to stand upright, walk, turn, and climb and descend stairs (ReWalk).

I know that you think this is all great, but how can I afford one of these suits. I, too, investigated the cost of purchasing an exoskeleton suit for myself. I was shocked at the cost. I would have thought that with this new technology that the price would be more affordable. I was wrong. Moving forward to the time I am writing this book, 2020, I have researched the many ways that I now can afford, purchase one of the exoskeleton suits. Today, there are many charitable foundations, veteran affairs, and many grants available that can help make buying one of the exoskeleton suits more affordable. I haven't purchased one, but I'm keeping my options open.

Another area of technology that I want to cover is the use of computer chips, electrodes to bridge the gap in neuroscience and paralysis. Since 1996, there have been many countries involved in computer chip development that will enable people that have SCI to walk again. More than 100,000 people just in the United States have electrodes implanted into their brains to restore the loss of function due to many different types of diseases, conditions, and paralysis (Team). These electrodes provide a connection between the body and the brain that has been lost to the person (Team). This connection between the mind and body is restored by the information fed into a computer chip that adjusts electrical signals into a wireless transmission

(Team). The receiver is located in the paralyzed limb, which will then pick up this information and change it back into the original electrical signal and stimulate the dysfunctional nerves or muscles (Team).

In March 2000, in Belgium, a 39-year-old paralyzed man was able to take his first steps since a car crash ten years earlier. All possible due to the technology and advancements in computer chips and electrodes. In time, technology and advances in medicine will allow a paralyzed person to walk upright again. Stay positive. There is hope!

Chapter 10

Conclusion

The goal when writing this informative self-help e-book was to keep the book simple, personable, to help others cope, adapt, motivate, and strive with their new life while being paralyzed. I hope this e-book was helpful in many ways to the person and their family that has been affected by paralysis. I included many personal experiences, information about myself while covering many informative subjects to help keep the information light, positive, supporting, and motivating. I hope that you enjoyed reading this e-book and will visit my website, https://www.facebook.com/MoveForward365/. Please email me with any questions, concerns, and ideas.

Stay positive, hopeful, motivated, and continue to Move Forward!

Appendix
Minimal Bathroom Layout Examples (Chapter 2)

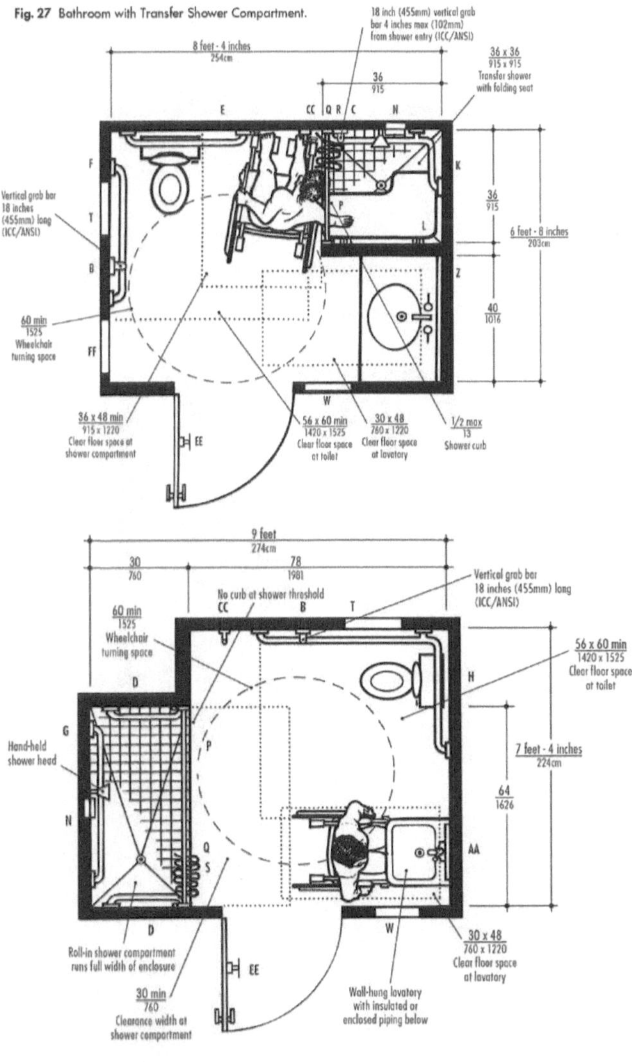

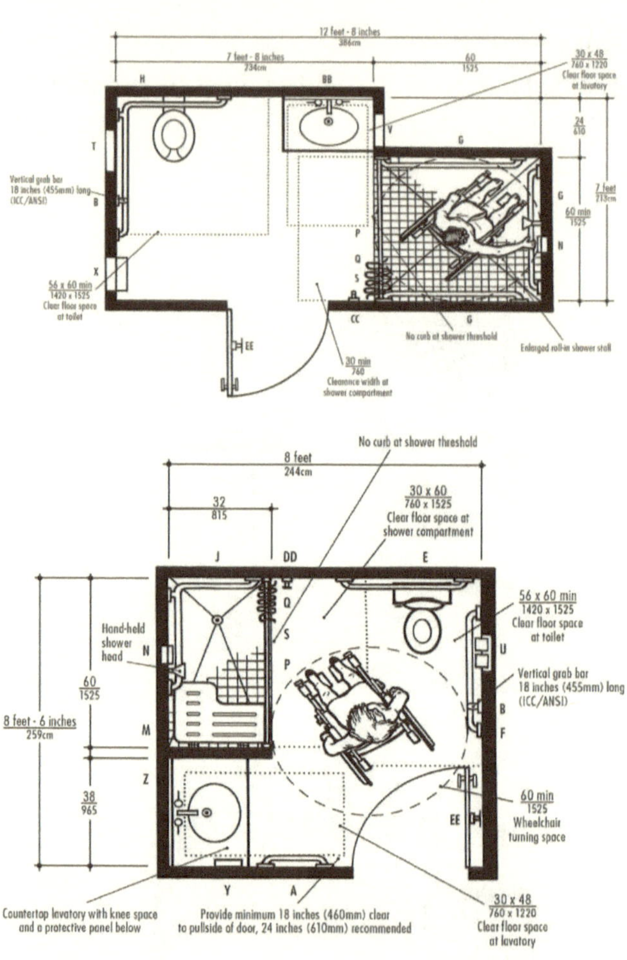
12 feet - 8 inches
386cm
7 feet - 8 inches
234cm
60
1525
30 x 48
760 x 1220
Clear floor space
at lavatory
H
BB
V
G
T
24
610
G
G
7 feet
213cm
Vertical grab bar
18 inches (455mm) long
(ICC/ANSI)
B
60 min
1525
P
N
Q
S
X
S
56 x 60 min
1420 x 1525
Clear floor space
at toilet
CC
G
No curb at shower threshold
Enlarged roll-in shower stall
EE
30 min
760
Clearance width at
shower compartment

No curb at shower threshold
8 feet
244cm
30 x 60
760 x 1525
Clear floor space at
shower compartment
32
815
J
DD
E
Q
56 x 60 min
1420 x 1525
Clear floor space
at toilet
Hand-held
shower
head
N
S
U
P
Vertical grab bar
18 inches (455mm) long
(ICC/ANSI)
60
1525
B
F
8 feet - 6 inches
259cm
M
Z
60 min
1525
Wheelchair
turning space
38
965
EE
Y
A
30 x 48
760 x 1220
Clear floor space
at lavatory
Countertop lavatory with knee space
and a protective panel below
Provide minimum 18 inches (460mm) clear
to pullside of door, 24 inches (610mm) recommended

Accessible Bathroom Sink Example
(Chapter 2)

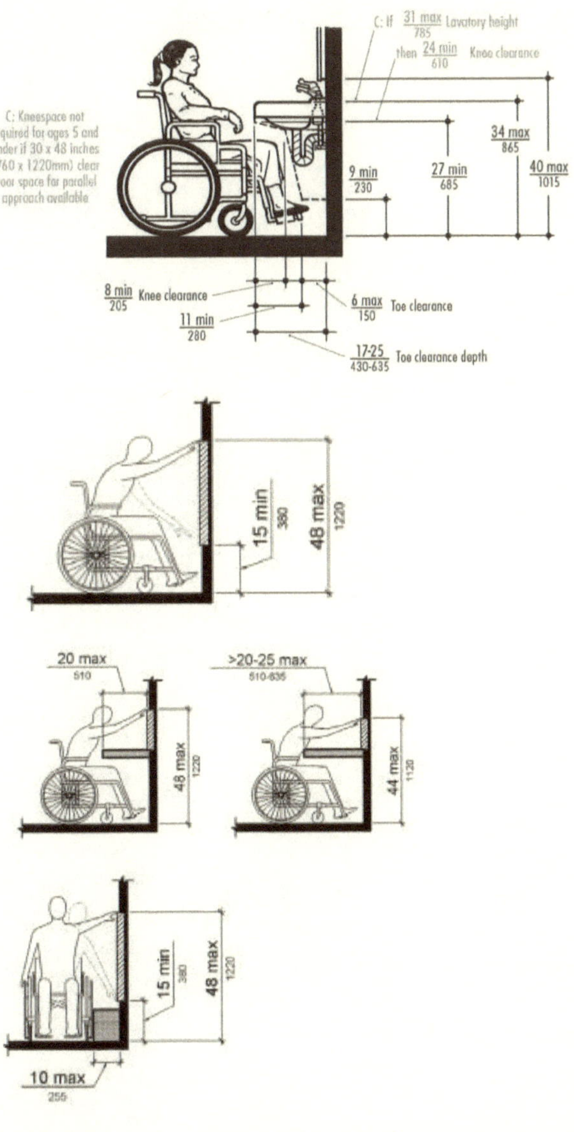

Adaptive and Mobility Equipment (Chapter 2)

https://www.harborcitysupply.com/

https://www.indemedical.com/

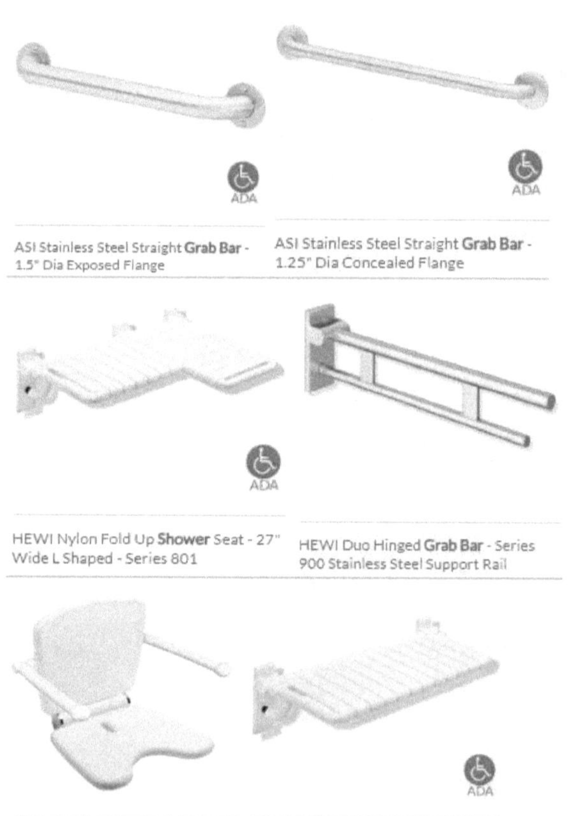

ASI Stainless Steel Straight **Grab Bar** - 1.5" Dia Exposed Flange

ASI Stainless Steel Straight **Grab Bar** - 1.25" Dia Concealed Flange

HEWI Nylon Fold Up **Shower** Seat - 27" Wide L Shaped - Series 801

HEWI Duo Hinged **Grab Bar** - Series 900 Stainless Steel Support Rail

HEWI LifeSystem Wall Mounted **Shower** Seat with Armrests - Series 802

HEWI Nylon Fold Up **Shower** Seat 32-3/16" Wide - Series 801

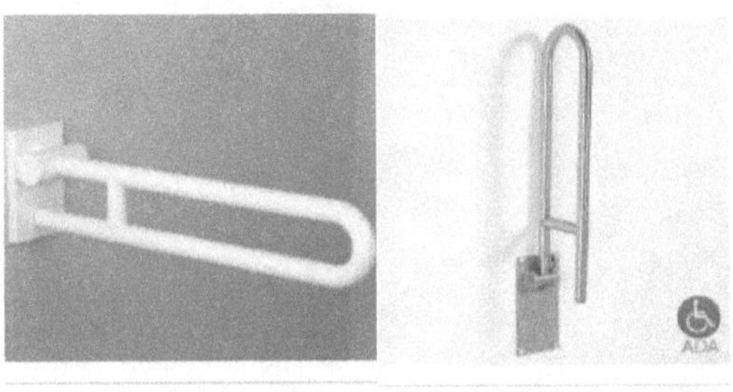

PBA Nylon Fold Up Spatial **Grab Bar**   Swing Type **Grab Bars** WC100

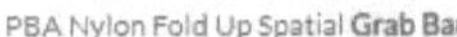

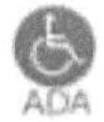

ASI Stainless Steel Straight **Grab Bar**
with Intermediate Support - 1.25" Dia

Hand Control Websites (Chapter 2)

https://www.sportaid.com/

Wheelchair Websites (Chapter 2)

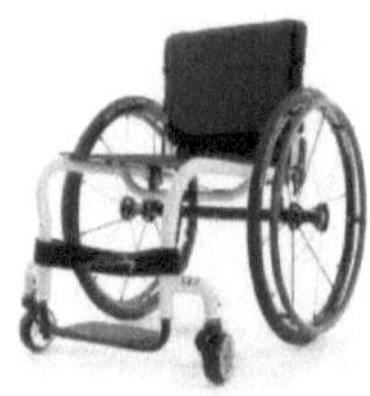

Q7®

QUICKIE Q7 combines ultra lightweight wheelchair technology, ergonomic design, and premium materials. Designed for superior handling, efficiency, and speed.

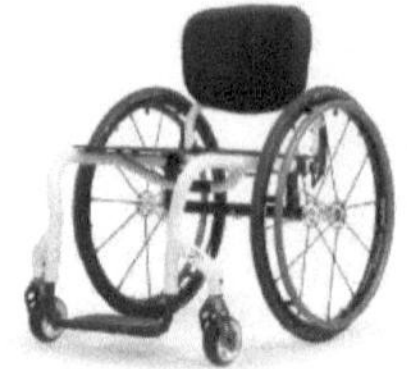

Quickie 7 Series

QUICKIE 7 Series combines ultra lightweight wheelchair technology, ergonomic design and premium materials. Designed for superior handling, efficiency and speed.

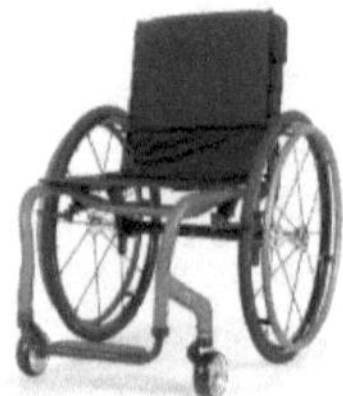

5R

Designed to deliver superior rigid wheelchair performance. As you and your environment evolve, the 5R's frame and components adjust to elevate your mobility.

https://www.sportaid.com/

https://www.sunrisemedical.com/

https://www.sunrisemedical.com/seating-positioning/jay/wheelchair-backs/j3-back

https://www.quickie-wheelchairs.com/

Medical Supply Websites (Chapter 3)

https://www.sportaid.com/

https://www.indemedical.com/

Adaptive Sports Pictures (Chapter 4)

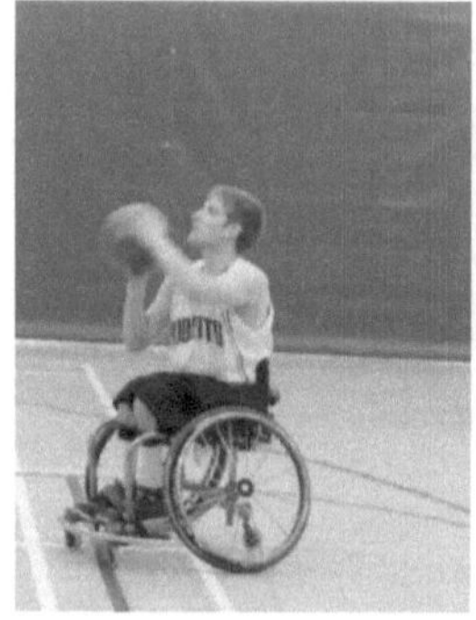

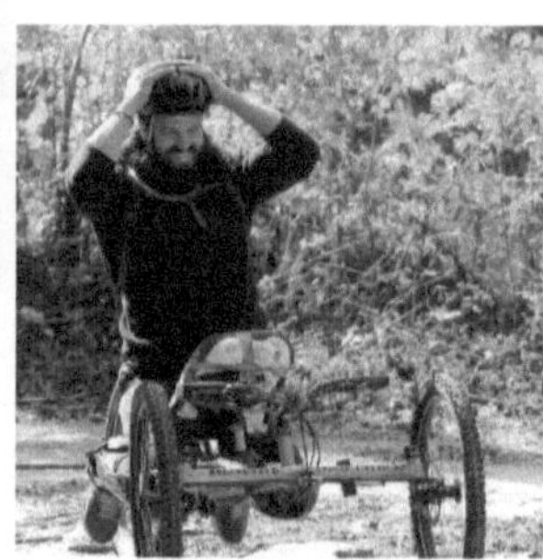

Cameron Gross   Jereme Gilbert

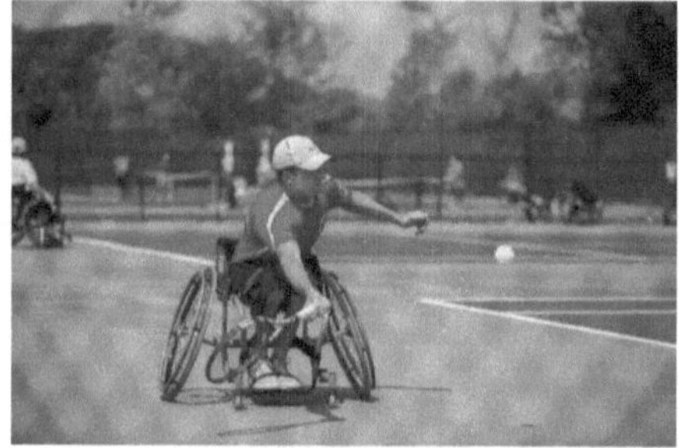

Taylor Wingate

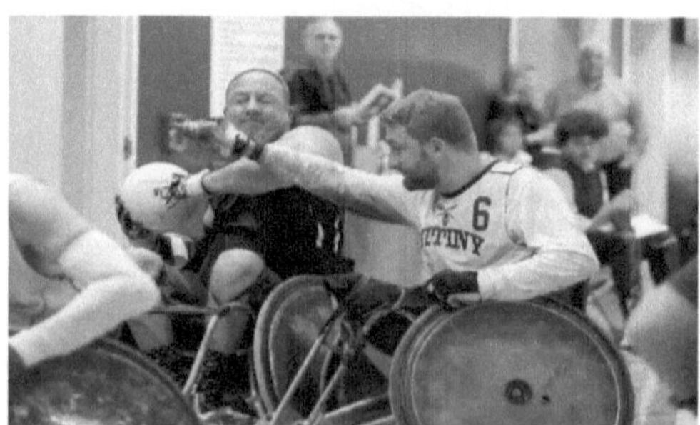

Robbie Parks

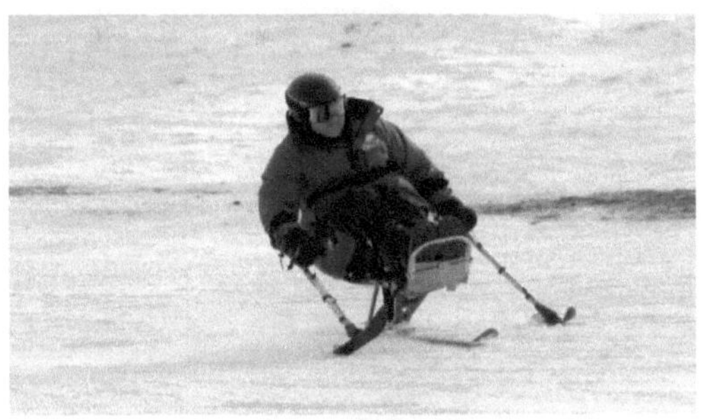

Robbie Parks

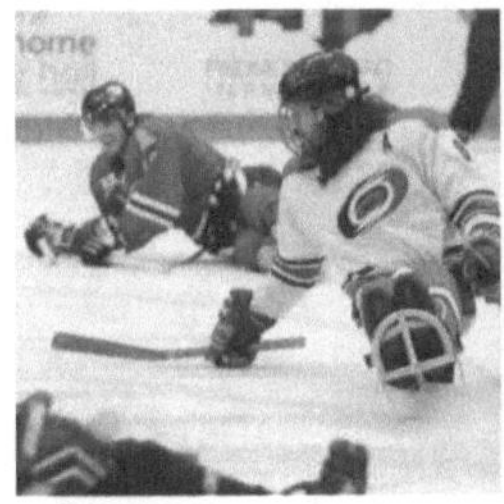

Jereme Gilbert

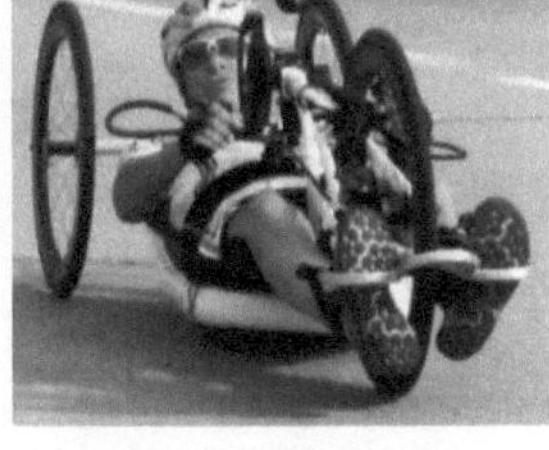

Brian Muscarella

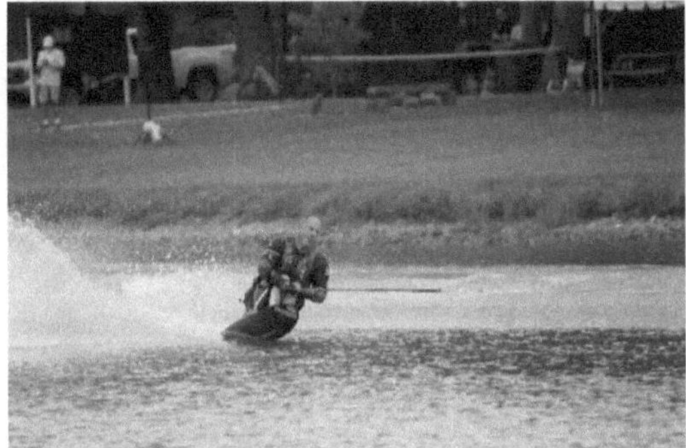

Robbie Parks

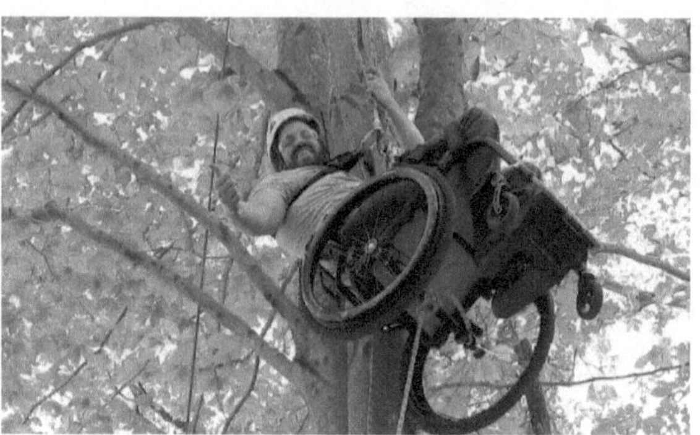

Jereme Gilbert

Additional Travel Websites (Chapter 7)

https://wheelchairjimmy.com/

https://www.airbnb.com/d/accessibility

Travel Gear (Chapter 7)

https://www.wheelchairgear.com/

https://www.sportaid.com/

Resource Websites

Christopher & Dana Reeve Foundation

https://www.christopherreeve.org/

Disability Horizons – Giving You A Voice

https://disabilityhorizons.com/

Information and Technology Assistance on the American with Disabilities Act

https://www.ada.gov/

North Carolina Spinal Cord Injury Association

https://www.ncscia.org/

Paralyzed Veterans of America

https://www.pva.org/

Wounded Warrior Project

https://www.woundedwarriorproject.org/

About the Author

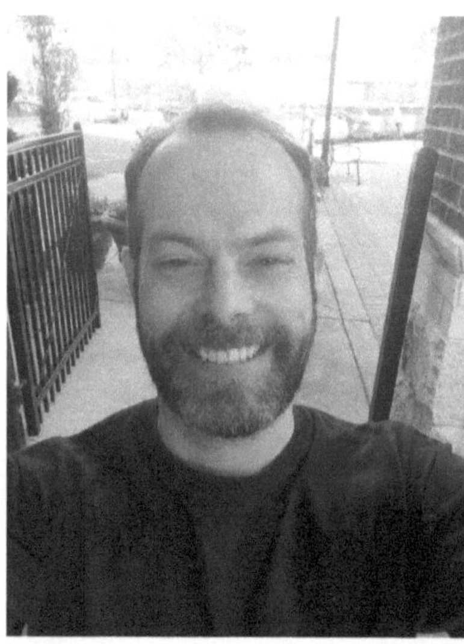

Matt Gustafson is the founder of Move Forward 365. A Facebook page that is focused on motivating and promoting a healthy, productive lifestyle for paralyzed people. He is an army veteran who served his country twice in Iraq. He is a motivational, informative eBook writer, has been writing employee instruction manuals for plastic manufacturing companies for over twelve years and will soon have two associate degrees in computers. He was paralyzed in 2014 by the autoimmune injury called Transverse Myelitis. He enjoys playing and coaching sled hockey, the outdoors, staying active and healthy, scuba diving, meeting new people and helping others cope with their daily struggles of being paralyzed. He hopes to get back into the water and enjoy scuba diving again soon. If you want to know when Matt's next book will come out, please visit the Move Forward 365 website at https://www.facebook.com/MoveForward365/. This website allows you to email, message Matt, post pictures about all things related to being an active paralyzed person, and more.

Coming soon, a YouTube Channel!

Other Books by

Matt Gustafson can be found at:

https://www.facebook.com/moveForward365/

(More books to be published soon)

Works Cited

"About Products - ReWalk – More Than Walking." *ReWalk*, 11 May 2019, rewalk.com/about-products-2/. [Accessed 3 August 2020]

"Health." *Reeve Foundation*, 2020, www.christopherreeve.org/living-with-paralysis/health. [Accessed 3 August 2020]

Mayo Clinic. 2020. Bedsores (Pressure Ulcers) - *Symptoms And Causes*. [Online] Available at: <https://www.mayoclinic.org/diseases-conditions/bed-sores/symptoms-causes/syc-20355893> [Accessed 3 August 2020].

"Reeves Foundation." Docshare.Tips, docshare.tips/reeves-foundation_58924448b6d87ff3898b47e7.html. [Accessed 3 August 2020]

Shop Catheters. "Intermittent Catheter." *Shopcatheters.com*, 2020, www.shopcatheters.com/c-coated-intermittent-catheters.html [Accessed 3 August 2020]

Team, Spinal Cord. "Microchips Showing Potential for Paralysis Treatment." *Spinal Cord Injury & Brain Injuries Resources & Legal Help*, 2019, www.spinalcord.com/blog/microchips-showing-potential-for-paralysis-treatment.

Vitality Medical. "Urinary Leg Bag: Catheter Bag - Urine Leg Bag." *Vitality Medical*, 2020, www.vitalitymedical.com/leg-bag.html [Accessed 3 August 2020].